Rucking Simple Treadmill Training

By Charles Miske

ISBN-13: 978-1983914164

ISBN-10: 1983914169

Why Read This Guide

You're going to want to read this guide if you are trying to lose or burn fat, but are having trouble making progress. If you're a runner who is injured. If you're on the treadmill and not making progress, or you're bored, or you don't know what to do next. If you travel and are stuck on a fitness center treadmill a lot.

In this simple guide you should find the solution to your problems. If not, check out the video and other training resources in the appendix. If nothing else, follow the link to ask me a question and I hope that your answer makes it into the next update to this guide.

What is Rucking?

To discover the meaning of the word "ruck" and by extension the word "rucking" you need only do a quick search on the internet where you'll discover a variety of meanings. Among them are the following, taken from Wiktionary.org.

• Rugby/Australian Rules Football: to contest the possession of a ball
• Fabric: crease, pucker, wrinkle in fabric
• Backpack: to carry a backpack while hiking or marching

It is in the context of the latter that this guide uses the term Rucking. In this sense it seems to be derived from the German word Rücken - "back" and the basis of the word Rucksack. While the use of the word rucksack is still common in some locations, generally we refer to it as backpack here in the USA.

Rucking is the slang term for carrying a backpack while hiking or marching.

Military units have actively trained with loaded backpacks for quite a while. Possibly as long as there have been wars. That's quite a while. It makes sense though. If your life, the lives of your comrades in arms, the lives of your superior officers, the success of your mission, the freedom of your country, and a whole lot more all depend on your ability to haul all your gear in and out of battle and still be strong enough, with enough endurance to fight to the death, then this is an essential skill. It's essential to train with a load similar to, if not larger and heavier than the load you would take into battle.

Military style units also benefit from this style of training. Units like the police, SWAT, urban fire fighters, wildland fire fighters, natural disaster first responders all need to practice training with large and/or heavy loads. It makes perfect sense to accustom the body and mind to long hours under heavy uncomfortable loads.

The rest of us though really don't need to train this way. Or do we?

Why Rucking? What if you discovered that simply carrying a weighted backpack while walking had the potential to greatly increase your ability to burn fat while simultaneously gaining endurance and muscle strength? What if it also could be proven to increase bone density? What if studies also showed a marked increase in balance and decrease in back pain?

It's true. All the above and more have been shown through numerous studies on the effects of weighted training, either with weighted backpacks or weighted vests. It's simple really. Put on a backpack loaded up to 5%, 10%, 15% or even 20% of your bodyweight and go for a walk. How simple is that?

Rucking Science

The Science Behind Weighted Backpack Training

In a 2013 study by the American Council on Exercise titled "The Metabolic Cost of Slow Graded Treadmill Walking with a Weighted Vest in Untrained Females" it was discovered that there was a marked increase in metabolic cost in wearing a weighted vest while walking at a moderate pace. In the study, subjects walked at 2.5 MPH with loads of 0%, 10% and 15% of their body weights at inclines of 0% (flat), 5%, 10% and 15%. Metabolic cost can be simply considered as "burning calories" for our purposes here.

The study resulted in a recommendation that walking at 2.5 MPH at a 0% gradient (no incline) with a weight load of 15% of body weight could increase your calorie burn by 12%. This is significant. It approximates the increased calorie debt that light running would achieve over walking, without a lot of the risks of repetitive impact injury that running often provides. The study went further to determine that walking at a 5% or 10%

gradient with the added load of 10% of body weight would result in a 13% increase in caloric expenditure.

The study summary suggests that in the interest of the lowest common denominator, walking at 0% with 15% load, or 5% with a 10% load would be the optimum combination to get the best possible results. In a scatter plot overlaid with a bell curve (statistics - argh) that might be considered to be fact, but the variations to stimulus that all humans carry within them implies that you should experiment for yourself to find out what your optimum load, speed and incline truly is.

That all being said, perhaps that's getting ahead of ourselves. Let's get back on track with our Simple Rucking Treadmill Training Guide.

The Ruck

Traditionally, the rucksack of lore, the rucksack that originated the whole thing, is a roughly cubical canvas sack with two shoulder straps and a little flap that flips over the rather rectangular opening and buckles closed. Perhaps you've seen such a thing?

In general, you toss in all your stuff, slide your arms into the holes with the sack on your back, and you're good to go. For the military this is probably about good enough as a description. Their prime consideration is most likely something like this:

The shape and size, straps and flaps, and padding all designed to allow a roughly 20-year-old in generally good physical condition and level of training to carry all the required gear the required distance at the required pace, while still shooting or otherwise disposing of all the required targets, pausing to eat and sleep, and repeating as needed.

Notice that comfort isn't high on that list of requirements. Obviously at a certain level of discomfort the distance and speed, and even the number of repeat cycles the soldier could endure would be negatively impacted.

We, on the other hand, needn't suffer unnecessarily, so for us the amount of padding, the shapes of the various surfaces of the pack that come in contact with our bodies, the various design features designed to carry our loads efficiently all become that more important. Yes, for some of us a training protocol of massive pain and suffering might seem pretty important, but in our protocol here, the most important thing to do is ...

Put some weight on your back and walk.

For many, if not most of us, this works out better with the right backpack for the job, that fits us the best, that allows us to simply load it up, put it on, and start walking for whatever period of time our own training allows or requires. If, only a few minutes into our workout, we start shifting the straps around, or reach back to lift the pack off our lower back, or reach behind our neck to pull the top up, or any other sign of obvious annoyance or discomfort, we might not get the full benefit of weighted backpack training. At worst, we might even reduce the load or the amount of time or distance.

Rucking Backpack Features

Let's talk about the basic elements of the typical backpack.

The bag itself could be shaped as a sort of rectangular cube, as a roughly pear or teardrop shape, or as a cylinder. Most are sold by volume usually either liters, or cubic inches. If you can visualize that a 2-liter bottle weighs 4.4 pounds, it will give you a general idea of the maximum weight capacity of the bag. This might not be a comfortable carry though. Your typical 50-liter backpack, even with all kinds of advanced support options, would be a rough carry at 100 pounds of load. For a more comfortable carry, assume one pound per liter of stated pack volume. This is usually closer to the designed load for that bag. Different designs of these bags could have foam padding between your back and the load. Foam might also be used to create a shape for the bag. This could be as simple as a round piece of foam at the bottom to support the cylindrical shape of the bag. Shaping the bag could also be achieved with bent wires or tubes.

Frames

There are a handful of frame options with backpacks. As they increase in complexity, they also increase in load bearing capacity. No frame at all is probably the simplest, with the lowest load comfortably carried. The bag is just a sack hanging on your back by the straps over your shoulders. Then, as mentioned in the previous paragraph, we have thin foam sheets to help support and shape the backpack on your back. Next would be a thin sheet of semi rigid plastic, often laminated to foam. This provides comfort and helps support the load, while still allowing the pack to flex and follow the contours of your back. Some packs have wire or tube hoops, usually around the periphery of the pack where it contacts your back. While not offering a lot of load support, they do help hold the pack in shape where it sits on your back.

The next frame system is often known as "Internal Frame" when purchasing a pack. Usually that's two thin aluminum bars, referred to as staves (reminiscent of the slats from a barrel), fitted vertically in slots sewn or Velcroed in the pack and typically resting along either side of your spine. These are often made of an alloy that allows bending them to suit the curvature of your spine. These can be incorporated into a system that allows quite heavy weights to be carried. Depending on the design of the pack, often up to 100% of bodyweight. One advantage of these packs for hikers on very rough terrain is that the frame rests quite close to your back, which allows for a level of control and balance not associated with the next frame listed below.

Finally, the classic external frame pack. This frame is usually a tubular aluminum frame that looks a lot like a ladder with angular support brackets. You might also liken it to a folded beach or stadium chair. It's curved to fit the shape of your back, but can't be bent to accommodate differences in shape between hikers. To allow for variety between users, the frame rests on foam pads or mesh panels and rests out from your back an inch or three. The main advantage to this style of frame is in load carrying capacity. Porters around the world can carry hundreds of pounds using this style frame. It's possible to wear just the frame and lash the loads directly to it. Such as boxes of freight hauled over mountain passes in the Himalaya or a quarter of an elk in the Colorado high country.

Straps

The chest straps go from loosely behind the neck, at about the level of the prominent bone in your spine (C7 as it's known), over your shoulders, and fastening to the bottom of the backpack, generally above your hip bone, the Iliac Crest. As it passes over your ribs at about the hollow between your ribs and shoulder joint, it can pass over a fairly sensitive nerve, the Brachial Plexus, and if it compresses that nerve at all, will cause numbness and tingling in your hands. This can last for several hours if it's not corrected immediately. The little strap across the middle, going between and connecting the two main backpack straps with a little buckle, the sternum strap, can help lift that portion of the chest straps off your nerve and alleviate some of this numbness.

Shoulder straps can be curved in various "S" shapes to follow the contours of your chest. Padding of various density, thickness, shapes and sizes can also affect the fit of the straps. All of these different attributes can also affect the comfort and load carrying capacity of the bag. Almost all backpacks use chest or shoulder straps as described here. In general, the thinner and simpler the straps, the lower the load capacity of the pack.

Hip Belt

The next strap to consider is the hip belt. Not all packs use a hip belt. As stated above, the thickness and complexity in shape of the hip belt contribute to the load bearing capacity. The least complex hip belt is a simple webbing strap sewn at the bottom of the chest straps and joined with a small plastic buckle. Add in some width, some padding, and a bigger buckle and you increase the load. As the packs get bigger and with more load capacity, the hip belt will become quite thick, and nearly rigid. The hip belt can be built into the frame attachment points, either directly to an external frame using pins and clips, or as part of the bottom of the internal frame sleeves.

The hip belt, depending on load capacity, will ride in the hollow above your iliac crest (hip bones) for a lighter load, or right over the middle of the crest for a heavier load. This optimum position will have some of the padding above, and some below, the bony crest of your hip bone. Some hip belts are heat moldable to allow for a custom fit where it rides over that bony projection. The hip belt is not meant to ride below this level, as it will likely interfere with your leg motion at the hip socket.

Tumpline

Finally, and I mention this primarily in a purely historical context, is the tumpline. This is a strap that connects generally near the bottom of the load and extends up and over the top of you head in a loop. With practice this allows you to place the bulk of the load vertically at the top of your spinal column. You'd be surprised at the amount of weight you can haul using a tumpline. Porters around the world still use this system to haul amazing loads. In fact, according to Wiki, there was a man in Mexico City in the early 20th Century who carried pianos on his back using a tumpline.

Rucking Fitting

Most quality backpacks meant for heavier loads will offer a selection of sizes in male and female specific cuts to help you select the proper fit with the top of the shoulder straps at about the level of the C7 vertebrae and with the hip belt riding either at the hollow above your iliac crest or right over the middle of it. There might be exceptions for specific packs and backs, but in that case a skilled sales associate at a reputable backpacking store should be able to help you make the best choice for you.

Extra Cool Features

Some backpacks have an extendable top. It's usually a tubular shape with drawstrings at the top and bottom. This could extend the volume of the pack to suit your needs, should you be using the pack for backpacking. An extended trip bag could have the top extended for a 60-liter load if you're using it for 5 or so days of backpacking. Then if you are only doing a weekend trip, fold in the tube and the bag now holds 40 liters. With such an extendable top portion, typically the top of the bag will be a panel or smaller bag attached with straps that can be extended or shortened in buckles to tighten up the top and stabilize the load. Unless you are planning on getting a larger bag for backpacking but using it at the smaller size for training, this might not be an important feature for rucking simple training.

Compression, or cinch straps are an important feature for us. A backpack could have cinch straps along the sides or even on the back panel. Tightening these straps compresses the load, tightening the bag fabric to make the bag the smallest size possible. I've used the compression straps on a 60-liter backpack to use it as a daypack and with the straps all tight it took up barely more room than a typical daypack. The tighter the pack is to the load, the more stable the load should be.

Hydration. Yep, water bladders. Most quality packs will have a sleeve or clips to mount a hydration bladder. They'll have a hole or three to extend the drinking tube outside the pack. If you're training outside these might be more important than if you're training inside. Inside it's relatively easy, and in my opinion much more simple to just put a water bottle on the treadmill in one of the little cups provided for just that purpose and use that. Why? Hydration bladders aren't much fun to fill and clean. This is even worse if you're using some sort of workout drink mix. Your sticky residue will clog up the tube and bite valve, rot in the bag, stain the bag or something horribly worse. I prefer to just use bottles, preferably wide-mouthed, even outside, just because I don't really enjoy cleaning a hydration bladder much. YMMV.

Which One For Me?

Let's talk about the different types of backpacks that we could use for this training program.

First of all, yes, the military or old fashioned 19th century style rucksack. The squarish canvas bag with thin canvas webbing straps. The classic that you might find in a musty old military surplus store. You might find it in your great grandfather's attic. You might be better off pretending you didn't find it. But if you insist, go ahead. Especially if you are already youngish and fittish and don't mind a bit of suffering. Oh, or if you don't plan on carrying much weight around for very long. That works too. In all fairness some of the group fitness style companies sell modern-ish equivalents and if you want to investigate those, by all means check them out online.

Next, we have the ubiquitous daypack. Most daypacks are pretty simple in structure and support. They're pretty basic in load carrying capacity. Most don't have any type of frame nor do they have support style hip belts. Though some do have foam padding along the back. Most daypacks also usually come in only a small or large version if even that. With these you could probably haul up to about 25 pounds without unreasonable discomfort.

The overnight backpack is a bit larger, perhaps 20 to 40 liters in size. You'll find these packs have better shape and support, better fit options, and padded straps. Loads up to 40 pounds are possible with these packs, though some exemplary models could go beyond that with relative comfort.

The weekend backpack is usually 35 up to about 60 liters in size. Now you'll see some advanced features in the hip belts and chest straps with molded and contoured foam and cut. This gives you the potential to carry perhaps 60 pounds of weight.

The extended trip backpack goes up to about 80 liters, has quite a bit of support with nearly rigid hip belts and very firmly padded and shaped chest straps. Yes, you could go up to 80 pounds in one of these and feel fairly comfortable if you select the proper size and fit it correctly.

Finally, you have the expedition backpacks. These are the packs you'd use for a trip on Denali or some other major undertaking. You'll find these packs going up to about 120 liters, and yes, that means you could carry 120 pounds in them. I know for sure, because that's the type of pack weight I carried when I was on a two week long advanced mountaineering training course in Alaska. Our group was dropped off on a glacier in the middle of nowhere, and the plane would return for us in two weeks. It was training for this adventure that led me to create the basic structure of this program.

Recommendations

My recommendation for a backpack for rucking simple training.

If you already have a daypack, or overnight or weekend backpack, that will be adequate for the beginning of this program. For some people the faster and simpler you can get into this and get started, the greater the likelihood of success. If that's the case, then hang in there and shortly I'll show you how to make do with whatever you have to make this work.

For others, the idea of going out and getting a brand-new backpack just especially selected for this program is the type of motivating factor that cannot be resisted. For you, let me spend a minute telling you what is most likely to help you succeed in your plan.

For most of you a weekend pack, something in the 40-liter range with enough compression straps in the right places to hold it together and tightly conforming to a pair of 2-liter soda bottles laid out side by side vertically along the back panel. You can visualize that, right? In this configuration your pack can grow to allow you to train at weights from 10 to 40 pounds fairly comfortably and with good control. In a pinch, or if you are willing to suffer some, you could go up to 60 pounds with decent results.

In my opinion, that's the best solution for a variety of cases. I have had a 16-year-old boy, rather light in weight, use a 42-liter mountaineering pack loaded up with about 20 pounds of weight for cross training. He's a mountain bike and cyclocross racer. For myself, I've used an 80-liter backpack loaded up in the 60-pound range as a maximum, and around 12 pounds for a minimum. There is no shame in announcing your numbers, either high or low. It's not a contest, it's just stats. We'll talk more about that later.

Weight and Filler

The backpack itself will have a tare weight. This is the weight of the empty bag. It will generally range from about a pound for the simplest of daypacks on up to 10 or so pounds for the largest expedition packs with the most weight carrying capacity. Obviously, you cannot go below this weight under any normal set of circumstances I can imagine. There isn't such a thing as negative gravity. Sure, fill it up with helium balloons like in the cartoons, but I don't think the volume of the packs would be large enough to allow for any reasonable lifting effect. Let me know if you can pull it off.

You will need to add weight to the backpack. This is weighted backpack training in its simplest form. Put on a backpack with weight in it. We don't really want to suffer though, so let's find some good options for loading up the pack.

I mentioned 2-liter bottles earlier, and in general, water weighs 2.2 pounds per liter, so we've got 4.4 pounds in a 2-liter soda bottle. Want to haul 45 pounds? That's roughly 10 x 2-liters. Ten bottles and you're there. Can you fit 20 liters of bottle in your bag? Your first thought might be that yes, you totally have enough room in a 40-liter bag for 20 liters of bottles. But bottles are round, and have some "wasted" space in the neck and base area. If you nest them like bowling pins, and invert the second vertical layer, it's likely to work. I'm just mentioning that in case you have a much smaller bag, like a 24-liter bag. That most likely would not work for 10 x 2-liter bottles.

Now then, let's pause for a second to remember my recommendations for size and weight bearing capacity.

A 24-liter bag using my recommendations would comfortably max out at 24 pounds, which is roughly 5 bottles. Plenty of room. Heed the recommendations and you'll be fine.

While 2-liter bottles are pretty easy to come by, if you don't fill them pretty much all the way, they can slosh around a bit, and if you are a really vigorous walker, it could put you off balance and even generate a wave effect. It might not knock you off the treadmill, but it can get really annoying really quickly. Fill them up.

One of my own favorites is large canvas sacks of rice. Sure, beans and wheat and the like will work just as well. Depending on what's in the bag, you can get them weighing about 5, 10, 25, even 50 pounds. You should be able to line these up along the back inside panel of the pack. If you were able to get a couple 5-pound bags of rice, a couple of 10-pound bags of rice, and one 25-pound bag of rice you'd be able to put together loads varying from 5 to 55 pounds in 5-pound increments. Oh, and substitute beans for the rice in any of those bags if it's more convenient for you. If you can find something like a food storage sale at your grocery outlet, or similar, this is probably the least expensive way to load the pack with weight.

I haven't mentioned till now, that the best place to center the effective load inside the pack is around your scapulae and below, and close to your back. Scapulae? That's the two cleaver shaped bones connecting your shoulders to the middle of your upper back facing one another. One of them is called scapula. They move around some when you rotate your arms up and over your head, then downward. If you just toss the weight into the bottom of the bag and plop it on your back, the load will pull down on your shoulders and cause you a world of hurt relatively quickly. I'm sure you know what I mean. How do we get the load to sit there? I'll share that with you shortly. Let's continue with weights for the load then we'll get to that.

Iron works well. By iron I mean commercial gym training weights. Weight plates, kettlebells, dumbbells. All of these work good. They are also quite dense, and can allow a smaller pack to carry a larger volume. I've used all of those options with great results. Normally these come in quite a few sizes from 1 to 45 pounds. The smaller the weight, the more weights are available. Dumbbells have the greatest variety of sizes. 1, 2, 3, 5, 7, 10, 12, 15, then in 5 pound increments up to around 100 pounds or so are fairly common. In plates typical sizes available are 2.5, 5, 10, 25, 35, and 45 pounds. In kettlebells it's usually 5-pound increments from 5 up to about 60 pounds. Yes, there are other and larger sizes, or weight increments out there. These are the most common though, These are the ones you are most likely to wander in to a big box sporting good national chain store and get off the rack. My favorites have been 5, 10 and 25-pound weight plates. I've also used 25-pound kettlebells in my own training. If I were to give you a generic recommendation for weight plates, I'd say get 2 x 5 pounds, 2 x 10 pounds, and 1 x 25 pounds. That gives you quite a few options for loading your pack from 5 up to 55 pounds in 5-pound increments. For most of us that's sufficient. Add in a second 25-pound plate if you think you'll be going much above that.

Oddball weight? You didn't think the bags of rice were oddball enough? Well, I've seen some pretty fancy plans to use 4" drain pipe with caps and hose fittings to make really big versions of 2-liter bottles. Or they're filled with sand instead of water. I've seen concrete blocks and bricks being used. In my opinion they're sharp and don't handle dropping and breaking well. Concrete shrapnel hurts. I've seen bags of shotgun shot, the little lead pellets. Bags of ball bearings work well, and pack nicely. If you were to go out and purchase these new, they'd be most likely more expensive than buying weight plates. If you happen to have a garage full of bags of gravel or buck shot though, use what you feel works best for you.

Filler is what goes around and between the weight, the sides, bottom and top of the backpack, and your back. Filler can prevent the weight flying around loose in the bag, hold it in position, and protect your back. Loose weight plates can chip if they clang together too aggressively. You've been warned. I'm a cheapy when it comes to filler. I use large beach towels, quilts, pillows, you name it. I'm sure you have something like this laying around your abode. Most of us do. One of my most popular YouTube videos is just me dumping out the contents of my 60-pound training backpack. I'll post the following example too, so follow the links in the appendix if you want to see it as well as other things here that are better seen than read.

Let me give you just one example of how to do this. Set the bag down with the chest straps toward the floor. Push a pillow down to the bottom of the sack and squeeze it in so it takes up only about 1/3 or so of the bag. This depends some on the size of the bag and the size of your weight load. Lay a quilt along the inside panel facing your back. Put the first layer of weight load in, resting just above the pillow and flat along your back. Flip the quilt down over the weight load. If there are more weight load layers, maybe you could flip the quilt into a little "Z" and slide in another layer. Repeat until you are at your desired weight load. Wiggle everything into place and cinch the top flap or pocket or gusset or whatever is at the top as tight as you can while still maintaining the bag shape. Do the same with the side compression straps, starting at the bottom to assist the pillow with forming a solid shelf to support the weight. Then finally the outside rear compression straps, if any. Now the bag should be quite stable, and the load should be located along your spine where it will be a good carry.

If you have a small daypack, without compression straps, and you know you'll probably rarely if ever adjust your weight, stick a piece of softer foam along your back. Put in the weight load. Then fill the bag with packing peanuts, bubble wrap, or whatever you have that can just fill the space. Pack it in tightly, then zip up the bag. In cases like this you can often just use one soft pillow and smash it into shape.

Let me know what you need here. Future editions of this work will include your crowd-sourced solutions that I might have skipped over, missed, didn't know you needed, or didn't even know existed. I hope this was sufficient, and with the videos, will make perfect sense to you when you are ready to start rucking.

Putting on the Ruck

Now that you have a fully loaded, ready to go backpack, it's time to put it on. Just toss it over your shoulders and slide into the straps, right? Not so fast there. If we're talking about only 10 pounds or so, that's probably just fine. But as the weight increases you'll have to start using other techniques or you risk pulling muscles or putting out a joint. You don't want to do that.

Up to a point, yes, you could pick it up, lifting it with the straps facing you and the bag along your side. Which side? Heck if I know. You'll naturally gravitate to using the side that feels most comfortable to you. With the pack straps facing toward you and the bag lifted and at the proper height, slip your arm into the strap and shrug it over your shoulder, across your back, until you can slide the other arm in. Shrug it into position and arrange the straps and fasten them. It's about that simple. A strong person could use this technique to set 30 pounds or so onto their backs.

At another, hopefully quite heavy point, you'll need even more technique to pull this off. Stand in a lunge position with the leg bent and knee forward for the side with the arm you'll be sliding in first. Place the bag with the straps facing you between your legs and close to your body. Grasp the top of the straps, or handle if your backpack provides one, and using your stabilized back, hoist the bag up and onto the top of your thigh. Let it rest there for a second, then rotate your shoulder in and under the strap. When your shoulder is well into the strap, hopefully at the full carry position, push off your legs to gently bounce the pack up and onto your back, supported by the shoulder under the strap. Carefully reach back and slip the other arm in under the strap and shrug the pack into position. Use your legs to help propel the pack into place.

This technique is used by mountaineers and expeditioners to lift hugely heavy packs onto their backs. I've done this with over 100 pounds in the pack. Oh, and if you do this with really heavy weights, let's all hope you've also done it with really light weights to get the technique nailed down, so you can avoid injury. I'd hate for you to just decide on day one of your own training journey to just toss 50 to 100 pounds in a bag and try this and end up in the hospital for a month. Just warm up to it, building up gradually over time as you become more and more fit and strong. Trust me.

Carrying the Ruck

Now you're standing there, with a loaded ruck, belts and straps all adjusted and fastened, and you're wondering what comes next. Well don't get ahead of yourself. Let's explore our new gravity for a few seconds. Hold your spine erect, so the weight of the pack is squarely over your hips and feet. If the pack is pulling you in any direction just standing still, you might consider shifting the weight around in the backpack, or adjusting your straps and belts. You will have a much better experience training if the bag feels neutral while you're wearing it.

Then do the same thing while in motion. Step to the side, shuffle side to side, step out in a diagonal lunge. Step up and down stairs or a box. You want the bag to ride as neutrally as possible. This isn't going to be perfect, so you'll have to adjust your motion a little bit as well. That's what this short segment is for. To allow you to adjust your own sense of balance, gravity, motion, etc. to the new weight of the pack.

Movements that affect you most might be rotation in place, bending or stooping to reach something lower than you, sitting or squatting. These probably aren't going to become an issue, but sometimes maneuvering around a treadmill, especially in tight quarters, getting on and off, adjusting the settings, or even reaching for a water bottle, can all affect your sense of balance adversely.

Obviously, the lighter the pack is, especially in relation to your weight, the less it will affect you. A 20-pound pack on a 200-pound individual will be almost insignificant. On a 100-pound individual it might be quite a load. If you start out with a light weight and gradually work your way up as you become accustomed to it, you will make all these adjustments automatically over time and not even notice the difference. It's true.

Mounting the Treadmill

The Rucking Simple Treadmill Training Program is based on wearing a weighted backpack while walking on a treadmill. Should be simple enough. If you've never ever been on a treadmill before, and just the idea of getting on one and walking scares you at all, let me put your fears to rest. It's not that difficult. If I can do it, anyone can do it. Really.

So now you have your backpack on, you've adjusted your balance and mindset to carrying the weight, and moving around with it back there helping gravity help you burn more calories. Locate your treadmill. If you have one laying around in your garage, or basement, or spare room somewhere, good for you. You have a lot less difficulty in finding a treadmill where you can easily get to it. Otherwise, assuming you are using a commercial facility, and they have a long row of treadmills, the less finessing and finagling you need to do to get on one, the better.

If the rear of the treadmill, where you climb aboard, is relatively open and easy to get to, great. Otherwise, if the aisle between rows of equipment is tight, circuitous or cluttered, you should probably just take the first available, easy to get to treadmill you can. If you have to navigate a narrow channel between the machines, wearing a backpack, particularly a very large backpack, that sets you slightly off balance, and sticks out behind you like a large bulky turtle shell, then yes. Good luck getting through that mess in one piece. Do your best, and remember that as you spin or rotate in place, your backside sticks out quite a bit more than usual. Even making corners you normally think nothing of, your backpack could cause interference with people or things.

Once you are standing at the rear of your treadmill get all of your ducks in a row. If you are using water bottles, carrying books, or publications, tablets or remotes, it's usually better to set them in their little slots, cages, frames, or shelves. Believe me, if you're already off balance, stepping up onto the treadmill deck, or platform, is a lot easier with your hands free and without a lot of extra stuff floating around to deal with. I just want to make it safer and simpler for you.

When you have your hands free, reach up with at least one hand and grasp the rails as close to you as possible. With one foot firmly planted on the floor, place the other foot up on the deck. Hopefully there is a place outside the belt where you can safely just stand. The surface should be textured to prevent your slipping off. This would be bad when you're wearing a heavy pack. If you are able to, it's best to put your right foot on the right side of the deck or your left foot on the left side of the deck. Whichever foot you start off with, set it to that side of the deck. Then when you are feeling all good and strong and ready and stuff, press up with that leg and stand, setting the opposite foot on the opposite side of the deck outside the belt.

Why not stand on the belt? For one thing, especially closer to the rear of the treadmill, the belts are not too difficult to jumpstart into motion just by standing on them. You do not want the belt to start moving while you are standing on them and not prepared. Now, hold on to the frame rails while standing, one foot on either side of the belt on the deck on the textured surface designed for you to stand on. Press the start button and hold the rail again. Most treadmills I've been on start off at something slow, like 1 MPH. Wait a second for the belt to stabilize, then holding onto the rails with both hands, one on each side, gently step onto the belt with your intuitively strong and dominant lead foot and be prepared to immediately step out with the other foot and continue walking. This sounds a lot more difficult than it really is. Another of my most popular YouTube vids demonstrates this mount and dismount process. Check the links in the appendix where you'll find the most pertinent extra materials listed.

To stop the treadmill and dismount, simply reverse this whole process. Slow the treadmill down to a comfortable speed. Grasp the rails firmly with both hands, supporting a good portion of your weight on the rails, and step off onto the deck with one foot, then immediately put most of your remaining weight on that foot so that the other foot is free to lift off the belt and place on the platform on the opposite side. Press stop and wait. When the belt stops step off to the floor with one foot while still grasping the rails, then set the other foot on the floor next to it and before you know it, you've completed a treadmill workout. Yay us.

In case you're curious, the reason I recommend starting and stopping the treadmill while you are off the belt is because some of them have a tendency for the belt to jerk or move rather abruptly when you hit start or stop. That could upset your balance, which is already slightly compromised by the added load of a weighted backpack. When the belt is moving at a steady speed you have control of the situation and can easily absorb the change in motion of starting and stopping since the belt is moving in a more predictable manner.

Let's talk about treadmills

Maybe this is out of order, but now is a good time to talk about treadmills. First a discussion about what a treadmill is, what some of the features are, and what features you might appreciate most in doing this Rucking Simple Treadmill Workout.

At the most basic level, a treadmill is a rubber belt laid out flat between two rollers, one at the front and one at the back. Really old school treadmills had multiple rollers, a rather short deck (the flat platform area between the front and back rollers where you are positioned over the belt), and were not powered.

Modern treadmills are powered, and usually have a longer deck. A longer deck allows a margin for error to accommodate uneven gait and footfalls. A really experienced runner with super good form has a fairly consistent foot strike pattern and can get away with a shorter deck. My "I'm a runner" readers might disagree, and that's all cool. Marketing for treadmills implies that since a real runner, in full on flight mode, sprint mode, etc. has their front foot reaching out 3' from their body and their rear leg also reaching out 3' from their body, thus necessitating a 6' deck. Anyway, just couldn't avoid sticking that in there.

Is a 6' deck important? The main advantage to a longer deck for us "really slow" walkers (relative to the 6-minute mile runners) is that if you zone out and miss a step or two, it gives you a second or so to figure out how to get back forward on the treadmill without falling off the back. I've seen people falling off the back. I've fallen off the back. Be careful back there. The back roller is usually the unpowered roller, and rides free, being pulled along by the belt. If you place your instep over the roller, you add a little bit of pressure to the roller and it can zip you over and off in a heartbeat. Again, be careful back there, both in walking and mounting/dismounting the treadmill.

Treadmills have posted weight limits. Usually somewhere on the treadmill there is a little warning statement, or sticker or whatever. Something like "Max Cap 350 lb" or thereabouts. This is significant for those of us who will try to abuse our weighted backpack training for a large expedition by loading up a 100-pound pack and hopping on the treadmill. My recommendation is to be careful to not exceed whatever it says on the treadmill. Now obviously, if you weigh in at 150 pounds and will never carry more than a 20% load, you'll probably never need to worry about it.

Most treadmills also have rails along either side. Some are coated in a textured surface and others are relatively slick metal. Especially if you are sweating and your hands are wet. For that reason, I myself almost always wear gloves of some sort. My own favorite is the half-finger cycling gloves with leather or synthetic leather palms. The open fingers allow you to use the controls easily. The palms offer some grip when you hold the rails. As I mentioned in the section on how to mount and dismount the treadmill, you'll be holding the rails applying a good portion of your body weight, which includes the pack weight. The gloves allow for an extra margin of safety.

Some treadmills have handles somewhere along the front for you to hold onto. These may or may not be effective for you. It just depends. Sometimes, especially while you're getting used to the treadmill, you'll need a little bit of extra security while using the controls or while reaching for the side rails in either mounting or dismounting.

In quite a few treadmills you'll find heart rate sensors along the handles or rails. This isn't very relevant for us, I hate to admit or suggest that. While my programs generally do have a foundation in heart rate training, the sensors on the handles aren't all that accurate, and there is normally no way to transfer the treadmill heart rate data to your apps, so you can track your workouts and provide accountability. You would be much better off the either wear a heart rate chest strap paired to a watch or phone app, or wear a wrist watch with an optical heart rate sensor built in. That's enough about that for now. We'll address heart rate training in more detail later. Let's get back to treadmills.

A lot of modern treadmills have quite a variety of electronics in the console. Headphone jacks, music players, internet, touchscreen browsers, are just a few of the more common. You'll also find a slew of programs to spice things up, and even programs to automatically adjust the speed to match your heart rate targets. There are treadmills with little memory card slots, so you can load up workouts of the week or whatever. Let's all pretend for a few minutes that we're not little bored children with no imagination, no direction, and no goals. Let's pretend that all we need to do is crank up a speed, an incline, and hit go for an hour. How many controls would we need for that? Speed up/down. Incline up/down. There you go. Hopefully your treadmill has that capability?

In general, treadmills I've used are able to be adjusted from .5 MPH to 12 MPH. Advanced models can go faster than that, sometimes up to 15 MPH. We probably aren't going to be running 4-minute miles with a weighted backpack. I might be wrong. Treadmills are readily obtainable with inclinations from 0 to 12%. About half go up to 15%. There are a few models that go up to 40% and very few that also go negative down to -6% as an option. That's like running downhill. If you are a mountaineer or serious hiker, that can be useful for the type of eccentric muscle training helpful to avoid soreness from downhill hiking. It's not a really big deal though, so if you aren't able to get into the negative inclines don't sweat it.

Same for extremely high positive inclinations. If you need sports specific training for steep trail running or hiking, yeah, it makes sense. Otherwise, remember that for most normal people, you'll get awesome benefits at 5 to 10%, which is typical on most treadmills with inclination controls.

Entertainment options

Let's take a half a step backward on this explanation and go back to electronics. Often times, and for me almost every time, you'll want to do something while you walk. After your initial exploratory "getting used to the idea of walking with a weighted backpack on the treadmill" period, you'll be free to enjoy music, books, videos, or some other form of entertainment. If you are using your very own treadmill in your very own dwelling, and are the only person to be doing so, then go ahead and use the built-in music player, or video player or whatever you have. Once you set it up it's touch-and-go and you needn't worry about anyone else.

If on the other hand you are using a treadmill in a public facility, I highly recommend that you bring your own goodies with you. Many treadmills have a shelf for reading a book that can also be used for holding a tablet. If you are worried about the tablet sliding down or flipping off the console, you can get or make some little rubber band or Velcro strap thingies to pin the top or sides or corners down and hold it securely. Swiping the screen while walking might be a skill that's easy or difficult for you, so adjust your needs accordingly. This is especially difficult if you need to pick things out of a list or somehow or other need more dexterity to accomplish. Swiping pages in a book isn't bad. Scrolling through a list of emails and replying to them would be horrendous. For me anyway.

The tablet screen might work out fantastically for you. You might also consider video glasses or headsets, which range from really cheap with tiny screens and look like really ugly 1980's style fishing sunglasses up to modern VR/AR viewers that look like they bolt onto attack helicopter pilot helmets. For audio, depending on your device, personal preference, and comfort, you can use various earbuds or headphones. At home I use wireless over-the-ear headphones, and dislike cables and wires hanging around in the way.

I prefer a video playlist that moves from one to the next automatically. Some of the streaming subscription services provide this feature. Music playlists are also a good option for those who prefer listening to watching while walking. Maybe you just don't care and want to carefully and intently examine the wall in front of you?

One thing you might want to avoid if you can, is to watch the screen at the gym. It's usually at a bad angle, with a bad show, with bad audio and outside your control. Ugh! Just don't do it. If by some crazy chance your gym offers the "Cardio Cinema" and you can finagle your schedule around it, and you don't mind working out completely in the dark from start to finish, including wandering around the narrow aisles between the equipment wearing a weighted backpack, and they have decent movies, go for it. Most of the ones I've used have been in really small spaces, packed to the gills with really old beat up equipment and played B movies from the 70's. Check it out in your local area though, in case my experiences were just really exceptionally bad and not representative of the genre as a whole.

Cleaning up

This is a difficult topic for quite a few reasons. Let me share a little story with you. I myself did a demo month at one of those franchise keycard gyms. You pay your monthly fee and get a keycard. The gym is basically unattended most of the time and you come and go as you please. Usually I do strength training wearing an old-fashioned type cotton hoodie, cotton sweat pants, and workout gloves. Imagine Rocky to visualize that. Not one square inch of my skin touched anything except handles, and that being the ends of my fingers. Signs everywhere proclaimed "Clean Your Equipment" and I'm like "Whatever. I've been in gyms for 30 years and accept the fact that people sweat on stuff and so long as it's not wet when I get there, I'm all good with that."

Besides, it's not like any of my skin is going to touch the vinyl padding, right? Well, I noticed that everyone there was doing circuit training. That's when you walk around from machine to machine doing a handful of reps on each one. Every now and then some fitness guru writes an article speculating that you'll burn fat instead of bulking up like a powerlifter if you do that.* So between each and every set, they would spend about 3-5 minutes scrubbing the vinyl. I'm not kidding. Scrubbing. Not just wipey-wipey. Can you imagine?

That's one way to turn a 40-minute workout into 3 hours. So what happens with me? I do my workout and leave. And get all these foul looks from the other patrons. So on my next visit I carefully look at the vinyl seats and pads from every angle, and see absolutely nothing. No mist, or condensation, or damp spots or anything. But still they glare. So I carried a little towel with me and a quick swipe at every machine and still, I guess it wasn't the thorough scrubbing they required. So I didn't go back. What a negative environment that was. In my case I had a handful of options for strength training facilities, and could select an environment that suited me better.

Now, if you're on their side, and require that a good thorough rubber glove boiling water sanitizer scrub be achieved on each and every machine on each and every set, I don't mean to sound like I'm making fun of you. We're each in our own place, right? Remember, with all my layers, proven by visual inspection, I wasn't leaving any trace of my existence. I was proactively keeping the sanitation levels high. They were sliming all over the equipment, then at the tail end scrubbing up.

How does this relate to your treadmill use? If you are going to be leaving sweat or food or drink residue on the treadmill, please take a few seconds or minutes as the case may be, and clean up after yourself. When I ride a cycling trainer in my garage, I wear a head kerchief, have towels on the bike frame and handlebars, and a towel on the floor under me. I do generate quite a bit of water when riding under sustained wattage on the trainer. I am being proactive. I wipe the seat and toss the towels and bandanas in the laundry. On the treadmill I don't generate nearly as much sweat, so I have towels over the front rails, and between that and my gloves, leave barely any trace.

In both cases though, it's my own equipment in my own garage. I share the treadmill with family, and they have their own cycle trainer, being a handful of inches smaller than I am and requiring a smaller bike.

If you are on a treadmill in a gym, rec center, or other facility, you'll need to adapt to the local sanitation standards. That might mean a quick wipe, or a deep scrub. Pay attention to the others, and whatever the majority do, you do. It's part of the cost of membership and training there. I mentioned in the stories of my own use, how I achieve my own level of sanitation, and it's up to you to develop your own.

* Circuit Training: Yes, there is a time and place for circuit training. It has value. If you know what that value is, and can explain it rationally, then by all means go for it. If you read a ghost-written article in a mass market print or online magazine, and decided that if everyone else is doing it you need to do it, then please, go back to the basics and start squatting, deadlifting, chinning and benching.

Getting on the program

In my bestseller "Summit Success: Training for Hiking, Mountaineering, and Peakbagging" and the online "Hikercize Program" derived from it, we assume that you've never been on a treadmill before, never walked at an incline before, and never carried a backpack before. The goals for that program were fairly extreme. Training for about 20 weeks with the end goal being to do a 10 mile round trip hike with a 3000' elevation gain and loss, in about seven hours, carrying a 15 pound pack. The weeks were divided into segmented goals for speed, mileage and inclination targets to get to the final target of climbing that mountain. If you're curious, check the appendix to find out how you can get on board that program at an unheard-of discount rate.

For this Rucking Simple Treadmill Training Program, we'll assume that fat loss and fitness are your goals. That means that over the course of your training you might not be concerned with weekly totals for mileage, virtual elevation gain (total mileage multiplied by percent of inclination), or total weight load carried. If you're a numbers and stats kind of person, and want to track your own measurements for accountability, even if it's just personal accountability, then yes, let's track all that. Check the appendix for a downloadable spreadsheet to help you track your stats.

With that in mind, the idea is to spend a few weeks getting into the groove, and stabilizing at a standard workout plan. Based on the ACE study referenced earlier, work your way up to 10% of your current body weight in your pack at 5% incline at 2.5 MPH. Now you've achieved a workout identical to the study workout. But you're not them, are you?

If you try that and break down, unable to move, with your heart pounding like a freight train steam piston, it's not bad or wrong. It's just where you are right now in your transformation journey. You might be just starting out in a workout program. You might need a few weeks to get used to being on a treadmill at 2.5 MPH with no inclination and no load. Then a few weeks to get used to carrying a 10% body weight load. Then a few more weeks to bump your inclination up to 5%. You want that all spelled out for you? I hate to keep saying it this way, but check the appendix. I wanted this little guide to be as simple as I could, and if I load it up with all kinds of charts it becomes much more complicated and puts some people off.

If you can just do the 5% incline at 2.5 MPH and 10% body weight load, right now, without holding onto the handles or rails at all while you walk, and not break a sweat, then what? Welcome to heart rate training. If you know your heart rate zones, and usually you can just calculate them or let your watch or app do it for you, let's check to see if we're in the higher range of Zone 2. If you're doing this manually, check for about 75% of your maximum. If you are above that at 2.5 MPH, then just enjoy the ride. You will receive benefits even if you're not feeling them immediately. Eventually your average should start to drop, and you can increase your own training load. Read on and I'll address that.

If you are below that, then let's bump up the speed and inclination gradually until we hit the upper range of Zone 2. At a certain point you might jump up to Zone 3, then drop back a notch and stay there for a while. If over time your heart rate decreases into the lower ranges of Zone 2 as you become stronger, then increase the speed yet again until you are back where you need to be. Read on and I'll address that.

Sports specific training or cross training might be good reasons to work into Zone 3 or (gasp) even Zone 4. That is totally outside the scope of this simple guide, so check the appendix for more recommendations. Right now, I'm developing a "10% Load at 5% Incline in 3 Weeks Challenge" and a few others, so go check them out. If you beat me, just get the newsletter and I'll be sure to let you know the minute I pre-release it to my most loyal readers.

Quick note on form and posture, since this seems like the best place for it. If you are stomping along at an incline feeling like you're going to fall off the rear of the deck leaning back while clinging desperately to the rail, you're actually not doing this right at all. Stand upright, in the front half of the belt, and swing your hands loosely and naturally like when you normally walk. It's not that hard. If you are leaning back and clinging it usually means you're trying to go too fast. Slow it down till you are not hanging on anymore, and work your way back up to the speed that results in Zone 2 heart rate training.

Training for the rest of your days

Okay, now you're on the treadmill, with a weighted backpack. You're Rucking. Simple, right? What's the plan? Well, if you are just doing something mildly interesting and different, with scientifically proven fat burning effects, then by all means, stay simple.

Rucking on the treadmill for about 40 to 60 minutes a day, 4 to 6 days a week is the sweet spot for most of us. This is simple enough to achieve without a lot of pain and anguish. It provides the simplest yet most efficient fat burning protocol without the potential for injury that running has. It's also functional. How many times over the course of your life have you had to hoist a load and carry it? Check out all the commuters on trains and busses carrying backpacks. Check out all the students with backpacks. Check out all the hikers and trekkers with backpacks. Carrying a weighted backpack is probably in your future.

As you increase in strength and conditioning, you can bump up the speed a little, or the incline a little, or the weight load a little. Unless you have sports specific goals, that's probably good enough for most of you.

Increasing the Load

Increasing load? This is where I'll address that. Most of us respond better with cycles or more and less training. If you want a set of charts and graphs and numbers, etc. I'll do my best to accommodate you, and if that's the case, then seriously, go to the link in the appendix and get the notifications email so you can stay in the loop. Remember that I love to reward my most loyal and on-the-ball readers.

Otherwise, if you want to explore this growth pattern, then let me share it as a little story.

Summary

I'm thrilled you made it this far in my little guide to Rucking Simple Treadmill Training. If you have any comments, suggestions, or even need to ream me out for my lackadaisical attitude about workout machine hygiene, please visit the link in the appendix and leave a comment or two. I'm happy to hear from all of you and welcome your input.

I'd also love your reviews. Both Good Reads and Amazon make it easy to review a book like this, and I appreciate all of them. It's the lifeblood of indie authors and is essential to getting the word out and sharing the message with future readers. Please, take a few seconds and make it so.

About the Author

Charles Miske is a fitness enthusiast living in Utah where the mountains are right outside the door for hiking, backpacking, mountain bike riding and snowshoeing. He is a certified mountain bike coach working with a local high school team and has been a certified personal trainer. He has participated and placed in international mountain running races. He is an Amazon Best-Selling Author with his most popular book "Summit Success: Training for Hiking, Mountaineering, and Peak Bagging" being the precursor to this work. He also has online training programs and workshops based on that book and this one as well.

Follow him on Facebook at

https://www.facebook.com/CharlesMiskeAuthor/

Follow him on Good Reads at

https://www.goodreads.com/author/show/7033020.Charles_Miske

Follow him on Amazon at

https://www.amazon.com/Charles-Miske/e/B0078CR5BA/

[If these links are difficult, follow the Master Link in the Appendix]

Appendix

Here we are, the appendix. I promised that I'd post more information here about how to get some of the media, downloads, coupon codes, and other important extras and bonus materials. I wanted to make it super simple for everyone, so I created a page that has everything you need to just click and go.

Some of them I want to share with you, and you only, my devoted reader, so please, don't just share this link on Facebook or Twitter, Reddit, etc. Okay?

Find all of the goodies I promise at this Master Link:

https://www.ruckingsimple.com/FinishedReading

Videos

I've posted two of the videos mentioned in the sections above. I have several more in the works, so don't be surprised if it turns out there are a dozen or more videos linked on that page. Bookmark it and check back on a regular basis as I add in any more that I want or need to share with you.

- What's inside a 60-pound weighted backpack for training.
- Treadmill Safety Primer.

Comments, Feedback, Recommendations

Have something you want to share with me? I want to hear it, so let me know. First of all, if it's a general public type question, and you want to share it with the world, you can ask me on Goodreads.

https://www.goodreads.com/author/7033020.Charles_Miske/questions

If you have something that you'd like to share privately, let me know at the form at the Master Link.

Hikercize Discount

Remember I mentioned a surprise super discounted rate for the Hikercize annual program? Currently (as of this publication) a one-year subscription is $197.97. Get it for only $7.97 with the discount code.

Why am I doing this? I want to reward everyone who had the initiative and drive to get this handy guide and read to the end. It's several months of very specific workouts on the treadmill with a weighted backpack. If you need someplace to start, it's a great way to go. This year I'm adding in several more explanatory videos and I hope you're on board to see the changes as they occur.

How do you get that? I'll email it to you. I don't want this code all over the internet. I'll lose my shirt if everyone uses it. Receive your code by registering at the link above.

Downloads and Programs

If you'd like the downloadable spreadsheets or the mini introductory training plan or if you want to check out and participate in the new and upcoming challenges, you'll need to go to the Master Link and register. It's free, so don't sweat it. Remember, I am rewarding those who've read the book and had the initiative to visit my page. I don't want everyone in the world to have access to some of this without first having read the book.

I'm also creating some Rucking Simple Training programs based on this book, some available on Teachable.com. The first one is free, so be sure to take advantage of it. You'll probably have all your questions answered in a heartbeat. If not, let me know and I'll make sure to make it available in future training material.

TABLE OF CONTENTS